Transform your smile and life
with dental implants

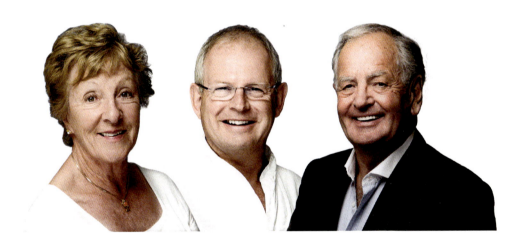

Tim Thackrah
BDS (Lond), LDS RCS (Eng)

First published in Great Britain
2015 by Elmsleigh House Dental Clinic
6 Station Hill, Farnham, Surrey GU9 8AA
www.elmsleighhouse.co.uk

Copyright © Tim Thackrah 2015

Tim Thackrah has asserted his moral right to be identified as the Author of this Work in accordance with the Copyright Designs and Patents Act 1988.

All rights reserved. No part of this book may be reproduced or utilised in any form or by any means, electronic or mechanical, including photocopying, recording or by any information storage and retrieval system, without permission in writing from Elmsleigh House Dental Clinic.

The testimonials in this book are the words of the patients themselves and have been reproduced, along with their photographs, with their permission.

A catalogue record for this book is available from the British Library.

ISBN 978-0-9934608-0-7

1 2 3 4 5
2016 2017 2018 2019

Book design and illustrations by Robert Updegraff
Printed by printondemand-worldwide

Contents

Introduction 4

Why replace missing teeth? 5

What tooth replacement options are available? 7

What is a dental implant? 9

The dental implant process 11

Bone grafting for dental implant treatment 14

Gum grafting for dental implant treatment 18

Replacing a single missing tooth 20

Replacing several missing teeth 22

Replacing all teeth in a jaw 23

Implant-stabilised dentures 25

Sedation options for nervous patients 26

How long do implants last? 28

Medical issues and dental implants 32

Factors that may rule out dental implants 34

The dental implant process at Elmsleigh House 35

How to contact Elmsleigh House 39

Introduction

This book is for people who are about to lose one or more teeth, or those who have already lost their teeth and want a better solution than they currently have.

I fully understand that losing teeth is a major emotional issue for most people. It is a problem that affects how we smile, eat and talk every day – all of which impact on our health, self-esteem and confidence.

Dental implant treatment is truly amazing because it offers the option of having great-looking fixed teeth again – something which really does transform people's lives!

The purpose of this book is to help you to understand:

- what dental implants are
- how they may benefit you
- the dental implant process
- what treatment options may be available to you
- how to look after your dental implants so they work for you for the long term.

Using this knowledge you will be able to choose the right team of clinicians for your treatment, ensuring that you receive the best long-term, top-quality care to obtain the most natural-looking and long-lasting results.

Tim Thackrah BDS (Lond), LDS RCS (Eng)

Practice Principal
Elmsleigh House Dental Clinic
Farnham, Surrey

Why replace missing teeth?

Replacing missing teeth is important in helping to preserve your long-term health and to maintain your ability to chew and enjoy your food, speak clearly, smile and socialise. All these things can impact on your confidence, self-esteem and relationships, which in turn can affect your life.

No one really wants to be seen with no teeth, to have gaps or to have to wear uncomfortable or unstable removable dentures.

Another important factor, which most people do not realise, is that losing a tooth removes the essential stimulus your jaw bone requires to remain a healthy, vital structure. Without a tooth, your body can resorb (re-absorb) the bone and gum in the area where it has been lost.

When bone resorption occurs, your jaw bone gradually shrinks away. The amount and rate of bone, and consequent gum loss, varies among individuals, but the process typically starts immediately after a tooth is lost and continues gradually for the rest of a person's life.

We have all seen, or know, older people who are missing most or all of their teeth, resulting in significant bone loss and shrinking gums. Without teeth and a healthy jaw bone, the face loses support, wrinkles become exaggerated and the jaw line is affected as loose skin sags. The entire shape of the face can

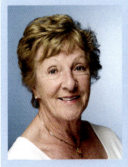

" Many years ago I lost four teeth in my upper jaw. My dentist mentioned that Elmsleigh House Dental Clinic was fitting implants, so I put myself in Tim's care and how pleased I am that I did. I was warmly welcomed to the surgery, my anxiety vanished and at no time did I experience any discomfort.

This was 20 years ago – now at the age of 80 my implants are as good as ever, allowing me to enjoy all types of food and feel confident when I smile.

Thank you Tim and Elmsleigh House staff. "

Mrs Shelton, Surrey

change; the loss of lip support and thinning of the jaw bone causes the nose and chin to appear closer together – effects that are associated with extreme ageing.

Many traditional treatments for missing teeth, such as bridges or partial dentures, do not fully address the issue of continuing bone loss and gum shrinkage, which, over time, can affect both the fit and function of a denture or bridge.

The good news is that high-quality dental implants act like natural teeth. They stimulate the jaw bone sufficiently to prevent it resorbing, help to preserve the gum and bone, and enable people to smile, laugh, talk, eat and chew with confidence.

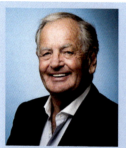

Elmsleigh House Implant Clinic has restored one of the most important qualities in life – the joy of eating!

I cannot overstate my delight in having fully functioning teeth and being able to bite into apples and carrots with complete confidence.

I had an accident many years ago which resulted in the loss of two front teeth. These were crowned with the available technology in 1960 but had to be replaced many times over the years. Eventually another tooth needed to be extracted and then a three-tooth bridge was fitted. Several years later a further tooth failed and I needed a four-tooth bridge which ultimately became loose. My then dentist explained that he could help me no further and that I would need a full denture for the rest of my life. No way did I want this!

I was aware of implants, began extensive research into the best way forward, and was fortunate enough to find Tim Thackrah at Elmsleigh House Dental Clinic.

From my initial consultation Tim filled me with confidence and he drew up a detailed treatment plan starting with a bone scan, jawbone augmentation at time of implant, and a continuous explanation of the necessary healing/recovery intervals in order to achieve completion of my programme in five or six months.

Every single stage was reviewed thoroughly with me so that I fully understood each treatment phase. Everything progressed smoothly with no pain or soreness. I was never in any doubt that my objective would be achieved.

My total confidence in Tim has been 100% correct and I am now able to smile and show a perfect set of teeth.

Tim has now restored my ability to eat anything at all for the rest of my life!*

Mr Rowe, Hampshire

What tooth replacement options are available?

So you have lost one, several, or all of your teeth – what are your choices other than dental implants?

Do nothing at all

This may be fine for one tooth, if it is not visible and you do not miss it when chewing. However, there may be some long-term consequences of doing nothing at all: gum and bone may shrink over time and adjacent teeth may move into the gap, causing future problems for the remaining teeth. It is worth getting the loss of a single tooth checked by a dentist to see if your bite will remain stable and that your other teeth will not change position.

If the missing tooth or teeth are at the front of your mouth, your missing teeth make chewing food difficult, or your teeth are at risk of moving, you will need to take action. So what are your options?

Removable dentures – partial or full

In the past, removable dentures were the only solution to lost teeth. Though they can work well, most people do not want something removable – a denture is not a must-have item!

Dentures do not stop continual bone loss; they often need to be remade every five to seven years as the gum and bone shrink beneath them. Each successive denture tends to become less stable as more gum and bone are lost. Dentures can make it difficult to clean around the remaining teeth, a problem that can lead to tooth decay, gum disease and bad breath. Dentures can make eating more awkward too – they often reduce the sense of taste. If they become loose and unstable, denture adhesive (a type of glue) is required to stick the dentures in place. This often needs to be reapplied after eating and many people find this unpleasant. Some people have such an extreme gag reflex that wearing dentures is impossible.

Dentures are usually made from a special plastic (called acrylic), but can also be made from a combination of acrylic and metals – typically chromium cobalt or gold alloys. There are now some flexible plastics that can be used in certain cases.

Conventional bridgework

If you have suitable teeth, it used to be common practice to cut down the teeth adjacent to the gaps and fit conventional bridgework. The adjacent teeth were fitted with crowns, and false teeth (called a pontic) were attached to the supporting crowns, filling the gap. This type of treatment is destructive to the supportive teeth. The life expectancy of bridgework, if done well, is typically only seven to fifteen years – a lot less if it is badly done or not looked after well.

There are complications in crowning teeth – about 20% of the nerves (the dental pulp) in crowned teeth die off over time. These teeth will then need further treatment, such as root-canal work. Gums may recede around bridges, which can look unsightly and may mean that the bridgework needs to be redone. If a tooth supporting the bridge is subsequently lost as a result of fracture or infection, the whole bridge is then lost.

Bridges are usually made from metal alloys and tooth-coloured ceramics, or sometimes from newer high-strength ceramics.

Adhesive bridges

If you are missing just one or two teeth, in the right circumstances it is possible to make a false tooth that has metal plates attached to it, which are glued to the tongue side of your adjacent teeth. This can be a good temporary or long-term solution. The main advantage with an adhesive bridge is that you do not need to cut down the adjacent teeth. You need to be aware, however, that stick-on bridges can come unstuck, and you will then need to go back to a dentist to have it rebonded. These bridges are typically made from metal alloys and tooth-coloured ceramics.

Moving teeth with braces

If you are missing just one tooth and your teeth are crowded, it may be possible to move your adjacent teeth to close up the gap. This obviously is a great solution, as you can fix both the crowding of your teeth, to improve their appearance, and close the gap at the same time.

What is a dental implant?

Dental implants are the most advanced therapy available today for replacing missing teeth. High-quality dental implants provide predictable, reliable and safe long-term solutions.

They have come a long way since the pioneering work of the Swedish Professor Per-Ingvar Brånemark in the late 1950s. He showed that if a titanium implant is placed in healthy bone, the surrounding bone will grow on to, and attach to, the titanium surface – a process called 'osseointegration'. Data and research from his work have led to a whole new branch of dentistry that has helped transform the lives of millions of people over the past 50 years.

A dental implant typically consists of three main elements:

The titanium implant – this comes in different designs, sizes and lengths and is inserted into your jaw bone; the bone grows on to it in a biological process called osseointegration.

The implant post – this fits into the implant and protrudes through the gum, allowing the final implant tooth to attach to it.

The implant tooth or crown – this is attached to the implant post and is the part you see; it is cemented or screwed on to the implant post.

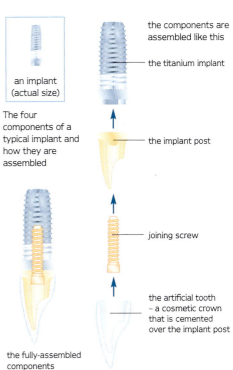

an implant (actual size)

The four components of a typical implant and how they are assembled

the fully-assembled components

the components are assembled like this

the titanium implant

the implant post

joining screw

the artificial tooth – a cosmetic crown that is cemented over the implant post

There are now thousands of dental implant systems used around the world. Many of them rely on limited research and have constantly-changing designs. I believe it is always better to use a well-researched and long-term, predictable system from a major manufacturer – a system that has been developed and tested over many years.

Dental implants are usually made from commercially pure titanium, which rarely causes an allergic reaction, though some types of implants use other metals. Some newer implants are made from a special ceramic (e.g. zirconium oxide), but long-term research on them is limited at present.

A dental implant can be used to replace a single missing tooth, and two or more implants can be used as support for two or three missing teeth. Four, six or eight implants can be used to replace 10 to 14 missing teeth in one jaw. Dental implants can also be used to attach, and stabilise, removable dentures.

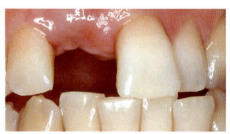

A front tooth is missing

Implants offer the prospect of having fixed teeth again – teeth that look, act and feel like natural teeth. Implant replacement teeth do not damage adjacent healthy ones. If they are placed well and are properly looked after, they are a reliable, predictable and safe long-term solution for missing teeth. Some dental implants have lasted for more than 40 years!

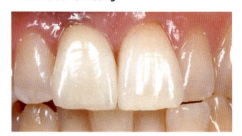

The finished implant with crown

These before and after photographs show an implant that is indistinguishable from an original tooth.

This tooth was lost due to an infection. Bone grafting was necessary to rebuild the bone that was lost.

The dental implant process

The actual process of dental implant treatment can vary and is determined by many factors:

- your overall medical health
- how many teeth are damaged or missing
- the health of your jaw bone and gums
- how your teeth meet and bite
- the amount of bone left in your jaw
- the specific solution chosen to replace your missing teeth.

Whether you need a single cosmetic crown, implant-stabilised dentures or fixed implant bridgework to replace your missing teeth, the dental implant process needs to be tailored to meet your individual needs.

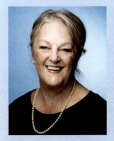

❝ I was referred to Elmsleigh House in 2002 when my dentist at the time was unable to address some serious dental problems I was suffering. Tim explained his recommendations in detail to me, providing me with explanations of dental implants and the procedures, timescales and costs involved. I felt dental implants offered a permanent and fixed solution to my teeth problems. While I was a little nervous and hesitant at the time, I had every confidence in Tim and went ahead. I'm so glad I did! Throughout the treatment Tim and his team treated me with the utmost professionalism, kindness and consideration.

The result was a total success; I no longer have to think about my teeth and what I am going to eat. I just take for granted that I can now eat whatever I like without giving it a thought, which is wonderful! As far as my treatment was concerned, I think it was absolutely priceless, I can't put a price on the result that I had. I can truthfully say that it changed my life, and I am extremely grateful to everyone involved. ❞

Mrs Sutton, Surrey

These are the typical steps for implant treatment:

Initial assessment – to assess your suitability for treatment and to determine the best solution for you

Initial preparatory work – to ensure that the whole of your mouth is healthy

Implant surgery – to place the dental implant or implants in your jaw bone, so they can osseointegrate over time. This may be done in just one operation. In more complex cases, two or three operations may be needed if additional gum or bone regeneration is required. Implant surgery is usually carried out with local anaesthetic, which means the procedure is painless; some people, however, elect to have sedation as well for these operations. There can be some post-operative swelling or mild discomfort afterwards, but this is easily controlled with mild painkillers.

Implant restorative work – to make the implant crown or crowns, bridgework or stabilised dentures, which are fitted on top of the implant or implants. Note: it is sometimes possible to place implants in the jaw bone and attach and fit immediate, functional, temporary teeth in one day. This will depend on your overall health, how much jaw bone you have left and how your teeth bite together.

Ongoing maintenance – to ensure your dental implant(s) remain secure and long-lasting, it is vital to maintain a good oral healthcare routine at home as well as regular visits to your dentist and hygienist for check-ups. You will be advised by them on the best brushing and cleaning techniques to adopt in order to keep your dental implants, and mouth, healthy.

Typical stages in placing an implant (shown as side views of a single tooth)

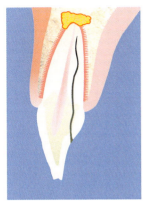

a damaged and infected tooth

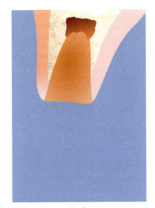

the tooth and infection are removed and an immediate denture is fitted

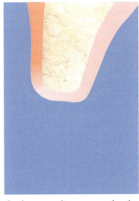

the bone and gum grow back and the area is reviewed

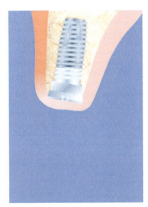

Operation One
a titanium implant is inserted in the bone and buried under the gum

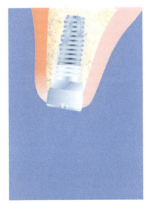

Operation Two
the implant is uncovered and tested and a healing cap, which protrudes through the gum, is placed on top

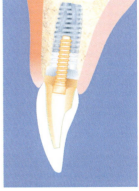

Final Stage
Impressions are taken and the colour of the new crown is matched to the adjacent teeth. The implant post is fitted and the crown is cemented on top

Bone grafting for dental implant treatment

One of the greatest obstacles to successful dental implant treatment is insufficient bone, which is usually due to bone loss from infection or resorption. Over the past 25 years there have been many different techniques developed for dealing with this problem.

Using advanced techniques such as bone grafts, ridge widening, guided bone regeneration and sinus lifts, a skilled implant team can increase the volume, size and shape of a jaw bone, which can make dental implants possible.

Bone-grafting techniques

Bone-grafting procedures are employed to help build up bone in areas where it is insufficient. Surgeons have a range of materials and techniques they can use. Their choice will be determined by your individual needs, but there are several ways that bone volume can be increased.

A bone graft

In this procedure a piece of bone is taken from elsewhere in your body and fixed where it is needed. Usually a small piece of bone is taken from your jaw, typically from your chin or the area around your wisdom teeth, and then screwed into position. The graft heals in its new position. After several months an implant can be placed in the grafted area.

For people who may need greater amounts of bone grafted, bone can also be taken from the hip, rib or skull. It has been more than 20 years, however, since we have had to use these extreme measures in our clinic.

> **If you have been told you do not have enough bone for dental implants, you should seek a second opinion – an experienced implant surgeon will have the knowledge and expertise to help you.**

Guided bone regeneration

Generally carried out at the same time that an implant is placed, in this procedure bone is taken from your jaw, usually in the area where the implant is being placed. It is mixed to increase its volume, sometimes with a synthetic bone graft material, which acts as a scaffold to help new bone to grow.

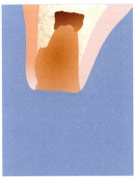
a tooth and the infection around it are removed and an immediate denture is fitted

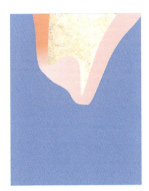
bone is missing after the gum heals

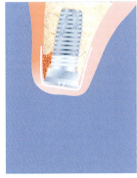
Operation One
a titanium implant is inserted and bone is grafted to rebuild normal contours

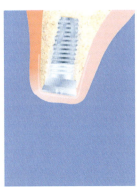
the titanium implant integrates into the jaw and the bone heals

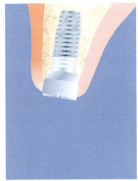
Operation Two
the implant is uncovered and tested and a healing cap, which protrudes through the gum, is placed on top

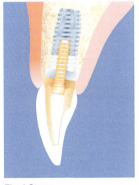
Final Stage
Impressions are taken and the colour of the new crown is matched to the adjacent teeth. The implant post is fitted and the crown is cemented on top

Sinus lift

The maxillary sinus cavity is in the upper jaw at the back of the mouth (see diagram below). In some patients the roots of the back teeth are found to protrude into it. If teeth below the sinus cavity are to be replaced, there may not be sufficient bone to accommodate implants.

It is possible, however, to rebuild the bone inside the sinus cavity to enable implants to be placed. There are several different ways that this can be carried out. Typically synthetic bone, or your own harvested bone, is added to the remaining jaw bone. To allow room for this extra bone, your sinus membrane is gently lifted up and out of the way.

Sinus lifts provide the extra bone depth required to support dental implants. If you have lost a great deal of bone, this will need to be carried out first. When it has fully healed, 6 to 12 months later, implants can be placed.

Sometimes it is practicable to do a sinus bone graft, a sinus lift and place an implant all in the same operation.

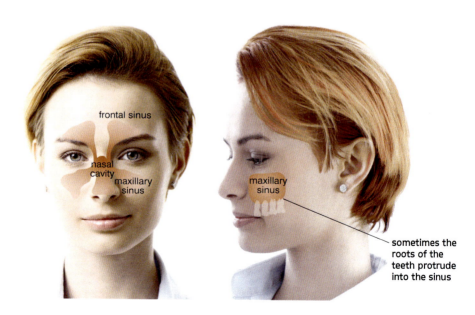

sometimes the roots of the teeth protrude into the sinus

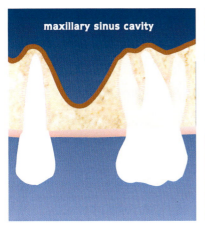

a missing tooth with insufficient bone depth to accommodate an implant

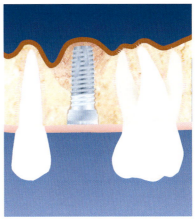

Operation One
the sinus is lifted, bone is grafted into the space and an implant is placed

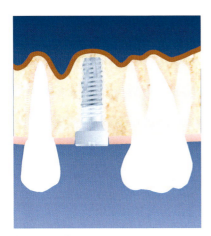

Operation Two
the grafted bone has healed, the implant has integrated and a healing cap is placed

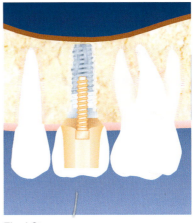

Final Stage
Impressions are taken and the colour of the new crown is matched to the adjacent teeth. The implant post is fitted and the crown is cemented on top

Gum grafting for dental implant treatment

To remain healthy, implants need to be surrounded by healthy gums. There are two types of gum in our mouths:

- the soft gum that lines our cheeks (dentists call this 'mucosa')
- the thicker, leathery gum that the teeth protrude through (dentists call this 'attached gingivae').

Ideally we want the dental implant to be surrounded by this thick, leathery gum.

Often when there has been bone resorption or infections have occurred in the past, gum is lost or is very thin. If this is the case, we will need to add more.

This is done by performing a small operation: taking a piece of thick, leathery gum from the roof of the mouth. This small piece can then be added where it is needed. The place from which it has been removed regrows new gum completely within several months. This area can even be used again for further gum grafting if required.

Where there has been considerable bone resorption, we begin with gum grafts to increase the volume of the gum, so that there will be sufficient gum to cover up the subsequent bone graft.

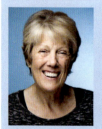

❛I broke my front two teeth in a sledging accident when I was 10. Over the years I had crowns, which were replaced several times, but my gums receded and problems worsened. My teeth didn't fit properly and I looked horrible. I'm a coward with needles so continued to put up with my teeth [but] I couldn't bite – not even a soft piece of bread.

I realised I needed to do something, so my dentist referred me to Elmsleigh House. Tim knew how nervous I was, and knew I hated needles, so he offered me gas and air, which was brilliant. I don't remember having four teeth removed and certainly didn't feel any pain – I immediately looked better when I came out than when I went in!

It is the best money I have ever, ever spent – definitely! I was so ashamed of my teeth – I would always cover my mouth and wouldn't even smile. Now I smile with confidence! Everyone at Elmsleigh makes you feel very very special. No one should ever suffer – everyone can change their teeth for the better! ❜

Mrs Quicke, Hampshire

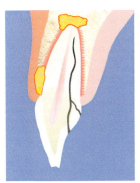
a damaged tooth with infection and bone loss

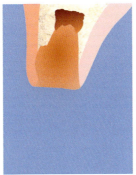
the tooth and infection are removed and an immediate denture is fitted

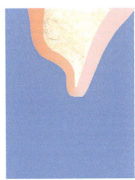
bone and gum are missing after the gum has healed

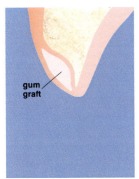
Operation One
gum is grafted to start to rebuild normal contours

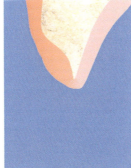
the gum graft has healed and the gum is now thicker

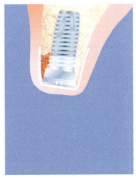
Operation Two
a titanium implant is inserted and bone is grafted to rebuild normal contours

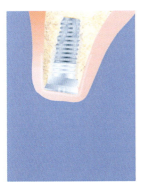
the titanium implant integrates into the jaw and the bone heals

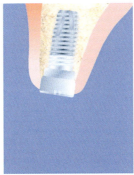
Operation Two
the implant is uncovered and tested and a healing cap, which protrudes through the gum, is placed on top

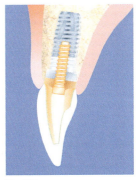
Final Stage
Impressions are taken and the colour of the new crown is matched to the adjacent teeth. The implant post is fitted and the crown is cemented on top

Replacing a single missing tooth

We see many patients who need to have a single tooth replaced for a variety of reasons, including:

- the tooth never developed during childhood
- the tooth was lost or damaged via trauma, e.g. an accident or sports injury
- the tooth was lost as a result of infection, decay, fracture or gum disease.

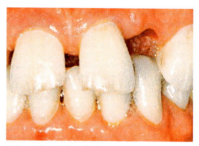

A front tooth is missing

A dental implant is often an ideal solution for the replacement of a single tooth. The adjacent teeth do not need to be damaged with treatments such as bridgework.

Initial preparatory work may be required before the implant can be fitted, such as removing the damaged tooth or adding a bone or gum graft to ensure a successful implant.

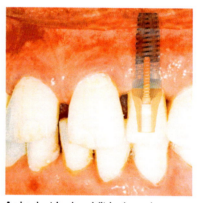

An implant is placed (it is shown here as a ghosted image)

This 64-year-old man had his front tooth knocked out playing tennis. He didn't want his other teeth cut down for a bridge, so we placed an implant when the tooth root was removed. A titanium healing cap was attached to the top of the implant at the same time, allowing the gum to heal around it. A crown matching his other teeth was later attached to the implant.

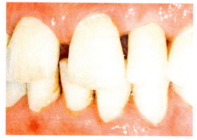

The finished implant crown

Where implant surgery has to be carried out in stages, a temporary tooth is made to minimise visible gaps during treatment. Temporary teeth can be fitted as removable dentures or as 'stick-on' temporary bridgework.

When the implant is ready to be completed, a cosmetic implant post and crown are custom-made by dental technicians to match the precise shape, colour and translucency of the other teeth.

In some cases, it is possible to have an 'immediate tooth'. A damaged tooth is removed, an implant is placed and a temporary crown fitted – all on the same day.

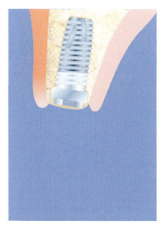
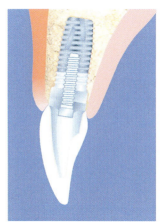

the tooth is removed and an implant is placed – a decision is made at this stage on the implant's suitability for a temporary crown

if the implant is suitable, a temporary implant post and temporary plastic crown can be fitted on the same day

' After losing my front tooth at the age of 14 in a dental mishap, I was left with not only a gap in my smile, but a gap in my confidence. The treatment at Elmsleigh was both professional and personal every step of the way. Despite the stress and trauma I'd experienced previously with dental care, I felt at ease and reassured throughout. Tim was able to fit my final implant before I left for university, meaning I could start this new chapter in my life with a smile I was proud of. Elmsleigh restored my trust in dentists, and I would like to express my profound gratitude! '

Miss Khan, Surrey

Replacing several missing teeth

Dental implants and implant bridgework are ideal ways to replace several missing teeth. It is even possible to use one implant to replace two missing teeth. Three or four missing teeth, however, usually require two or three implants to create sufficient support for their bridgework.

As a general rule, we prefer to use one implant for every other missing tooth; of course there are exceptions to this. We do, however, advise one implant for each missing tooth when treating patients who grind or clench their teeth, because grinding puts a great deal of force on to the implants.

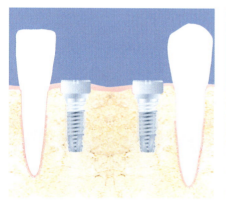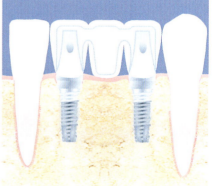

Two implants are placed in the jaw and a tailor-made, three-tooth implant bridge is fitted on to them.

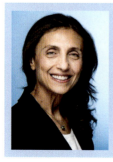

*From the moment I walked into reception, and in every moment with every person that I have dealt with at Elmsleigh House, I have been totally impressed.

From Tim Thackrah, my dentist, a breath of fresh air whose ethos of professionalism and care is stamped everywhere on the practice, to John Hubbard, the ceramist whose dental creations are precise works of art.

I thank you for every minute you have spent to ensure that I am well treated and happy with the results.*

Mrs Turner, Hertfordshire

Replacing all teeth in a jaw

In the past, the only option for someone who had lost all their teeth was to spend the rest of their life with a full set of removable dentures. This is also the future for people whose teeth have all been affected by advanced gum disease, severe dental decay or a combination of these factors. Not an ideal result!

Many people suffer with dentures for most of their lives. Dental implants, however, provide an amazing life-changing alternative.

Using only four to eight dental implants to secure a fixed implant bridge, 10 to 14 teeth can be replaced in each jaw. An implant-retained bridge can be made from many different materials.

There are two basic approaches:

Approach One – Delayed

Treatment is usually divided into four phases, over a four- to six-month period:

- removal of any teeth and infection in the bone and the fitting of an immediate denture, followed by a healing period – typically two to four months
- placing the dental implants in the bone under the gum
- uncovering and testing the implants
- making and fitting the implant bridgework.

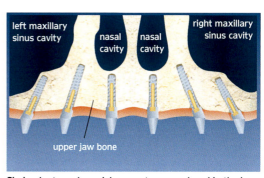

Six implants and special connectors are placed in the jaw

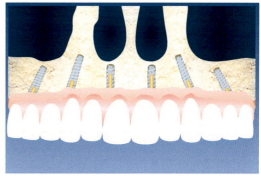

A fixed implant bridge is fitted on to the implants and connectors

Approach Two - Immediate

It is possible for some people to have immediate teeth by:

- removing any teeth that cannot be saved and immediately fitting dental implants and a transitional temporary bridge – all on the same day

- then after a healing period – typically three to six months – the final implant bridgework is made and fitted, which means patients do not have to put up with a removable denture.

The various treatment options that are available to you will depend upon your individual health and physical condition, which need to be carefully assessed. It should be noted that some patients may require bone- and gum-grafting procedures before we can begin any treatment.

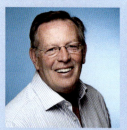

❝I thought I would give you a quick summary ten days in from replacing my teeth with immediate implants. The conclusion is quite simple 'One of the best things I have ever done. Feel great and look a lot better'!

I did experience swelling and soreness afterwards, which I alleviated with ice packs and rest. However, by the time I returned to work five days after the operation, I could not stop smiling with a new set of gnashers! For ten years I had always hidden my teeth. They have never appeared in a photo as I was so embarrassed about them.

I'm having my first check-up this week. The stitches are starting to dissolve. No swelling, no pain. I'm just so pleased I had it done – and wish I had done it years ago. Expensive but worth every penny. And as I said earlier, Tim is fantastic and gives me every confidence!❞

Mr Grant, Surrey

Implant-stabilised dentures

Implant-fixed bridgework (discussed on the previous pages) may not provide the best solution for people who have lost their teeth years ago, or may have lost a significant amount of jaw bone and gum. It also may not be possible to design a bridge that provides adequate support for the lips or one that is easily cleaned. Some patients may not have a budget that can stretch to a fixed-bridge solution. In all instances, an implant-stabilised denture can offer an effective solution to the replacement of missing teeth.

Stabilisation with dental implants is one of the most cost-effective ways to secure a denture that is loose. Special connectors attach to the implants, anchoring your denture to stop it moving. Your denture will remain secure and will not suddenly dislodge when eating or talking. You will no longer need a messy denture adhesive.

Problems with loose lower dentures are more common than with upper ones. To secure a lower denture that moves, we usually place two dental implants at the front of the lower jaw to fix it firmly.

To stabilise a loose upper denture, our normal practice is to use three or four implants – as this bone is less dense – and link them together with a metal framework to which a denture can be attached.

If sufficient support can be achieved from four or more implants in the upper jaw, we are often able to design a new denture so that the roof of the mouth is not covered by it. This helps enormously to increase the taste and appeal of food.

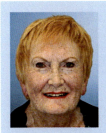

I had worn a partial denture for years, which of course had support from adjoining teeth, but that had had an adverse affect on my own teeth and it started to become quite loose. I thought my dental technician might be able to help me. He had a look at my mouth and decided that I could possibly do with implants. My first reaction was but surely I'm too old for that and he said no, not at all, you are healthy. He introduced me to Elmsleigh House Dental Clinic and we took it from there. In March I finally had my new denture. It was very stable and within a couple of days I felt like I had been using it forever.

Mrs Pullen, Hampshire

Sedation options for nervous patients

The thought of having a surgical operation for dental implant treatment can be daunting, especially if you are already anxious about dental treatment. However, the good news is that there are various options to help.

All implant patients are given a local anaesthetic for treatment, which means they do not feel any pain or discomfort. However, in addition, the following options are available.

Inhalation sedation

This is the mildest of the sedation options. It is more commonly called 'gas and air'. It has excellent pain-killing properties and can also reduce the gag reflex – the feeling of choking or feeling sick. A mixture of oxygen and nitrous oxide is delivered through a nosepiece. Because the sedative effect ends when you stop inhaling the gas mixture, 20 to 30 minutes later you will be able to drive safely or travel home unaccompanied.

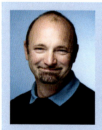

As a child I was very anxious about going to the dentist as my parents never went. This fear has stayed with me, with a feeling that I wanted to be knocked out to even go to the dentists! Over the years I have had many problems with my teeth, meaning that I needed implants.

When I came to see Tim, his explanation of the process still left me with nervousness about how much pain I would have. I was very nervous on the morning of the implants. Once I had the fluid Tim gave me [oral sedation], I felt great! From that point on I didn't feel a thing!

Tim's calmness and experience with dealing with nervous patients is fantastic! When I went home I had no problems with the implants, and am so pleased I have had this done.

So if anyone is anxious about dental treatment, I want to tell them not to worry as Tim's calmness and experience is fantastic! After years of having problems with my teeth I can see that by the end of the year I will have finished my implant treatment and have new teeth that will last. I now no longer hide my smile and laugh with my hand, and am delighted with my new teeth! Thanks to Tim and the team!

Mr Chandler, Hampshire

Oral sedation

If you prefer to be drowsy during treatment, a rapid-acting, mild, liquid sedative could be the best option.

Intravenous sedation

If you are very nervous and prefer a stronger sedation during treatment, you can choose intravenous sedation. This will make you unaware of treatment; you remain conscious and breathe on your own, unlike a general anaesthetic administered in hospital.

> **With either the oral or intravenous method your state of sedation is carefully maintained and monitored throughout treatment. The effects, however, will last beyond the duration of the treatment so you will need an adult to accompany you home. You will not be able to take public transport home or to drive for 24 hours after treatment, so please plan ahead.**

General anaesthetic

It is rare that a general anaesthetic is needed with modern sedation techniques, but in extreme cases this may be the only solution. It is safest to have this carried out in a hospital environment. The last patient that needed general anaesthesia in our clinic was operated on in 1989. We haven't needed to do this since.

How long do implants last?

Patients naturally want to know how long their implants will last. For most people, implant treatment is a very successful long-lasting solution. Many studies show that over 90% of implants are still functioning 20 years after they were placed. Some dental implants have even lasted for more than 40 years! We have patients in our clinic who had dental implants more than 28 years ago and are still enjoying their replacement teeth without requiring any further work.

In the same way that crowns and fillings wear out and need to be replaced, implant crowns and bridgework on top of the implants may wear or break over time. The good news is that these external parts can easily be removed, repaired and renewed while the implants remain firmly fixed in your jaw bone.

The key to long-term success is excellent daily home care, avoid smoking and have good long-term professional monitoring.

There are several risk factors, but with care they can be minimised.

Gum disease

The bacteria (dental plaque) that grows on our teeth is the cause of tooth decay and gum disease. Bacterial poisons, and the reaction of your body to them, cause localised inflammation in your gums and supporting bone. Over time this can lead to the destruction of the fibres that attach your teeth to the supporting jaw bone, with subsequent loss of bone. This process eventually leads to the loss of the affected teeth – it is called periodontal disease, and is the major reason why people lose their teeth. Some people are genetically more prone to gum problems, so have to be even more attentive to home care and cleaning of their teeth.

The bacteria that cause gum disease can also affect dental implants, so it is important that gum disease is treated and your mouth is healthy before embarking on implant treatment. Research shows that patients with a history of gum disease are more prone to gum problems around their implants – they need to take extra care looking after their implants.

Smoking

Smoking does not mean you cannot have implants. It does, however, increase the severity of gum disease, and smokers do not heal as well as non-smokers after surgery. This can be an issue when patients need extensive bone- or gum-grafting procedures. Smokers do not respond as well to gum treatment and often have more gum problems. Quitting or reducing smoking will greatly increase your overall health and improve the long-term success of your treatment.

Peri-implantitis

Dental implants do not decay like teeth; but the supporting bone can be lost around the implant in a process called peri-implantitis. This is a growing problem. Research has shown that some implant systems are more susceptible to this problem than others. A well-researched and proven implant system, used in conjunction with thorough daily cleaning, has been shown to significantly reduce the risk of developing peri-implantitis.

To avoid peri-implantitis it is imperative that:

- the implant is meticulously cleaned every day using a toothbrush as well as interdental brushes and/or dental floss
- you avoid smoking
- gum disease is carefully monitored and kept under control
- the implant protrudes through thick, leathery gum
- the implant is placed by an experienced implant dentist who ensures it is positioned well in the bone
- the implant is made of high-quality components that have at least a 10-year record of success.

It is far better to prevent than to treat peri-implantitis, which is difficult to deal with and may often require localised surgery and additional regular professional maintenance. If the problem progresses, the implant will need to be removed before too much surrounding bone is lost. In these cases, if caught early a new implant can usually be successfully placed.

Increasingly, we are seeing more patients with implants that are failing or have failed as a result of peri-implantitis. As more implants are being placed, poorly researched implant systems are being used more often. In addition, less-experienced dentists are placing implants in patients who have untreated gum disease. Patients are sometimes not shown how to clean their implants properly or they simply do not bother to look after their implants.

The risks of developing peri-implantitis
There are many factors that can affect your chances of getting peri-implantitis and losing your implants – here are some of them.

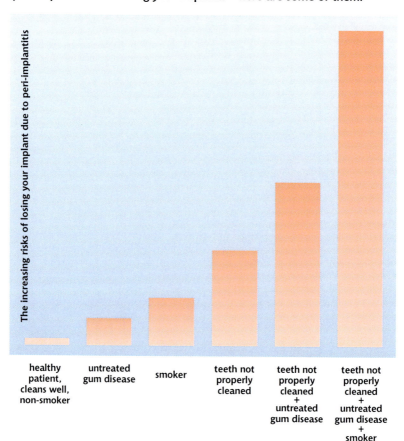

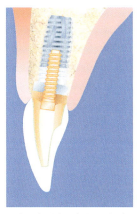 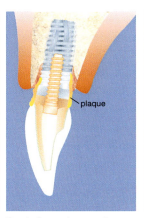 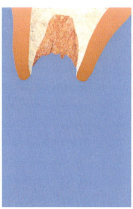

an implant has integrated – its health is maintained by good cleaning

if not cleaned properly, plaque begins to form. The gums become infected and the bone begins to erode

finally the implant falls out – bone and gum are lost as well

I cannot emphasise enough how important it is to:

- protect your implant investment by cleaning them thoroughly
- avoid smoking
- have regular hygienist appointments
- have your implants regularly monitored by a professional.

Teeth grinding and breaking implants

This does not apply to everyone but some patients grind and clench their teeth – a condition called bruxing. These patients apply abnormal forces to their teeth when grinding, mostly during the night; they often wear their teeth down or fracture them, as well as damaging their crowns, bridges or dental implants. These patients are at risk of fracturing an implant. Wearing a tooth guard at night seems to be the best solution to minimise this problem.

Medical issues and dental implants

For the majority of healthy patients there are no issues or special precautions relating to dental implant treatment.

There are though some medical conditions and medications that do have an impact on dental implant treatment. Careful management, however, can minimise any risks or complications.

Diabetes

Implants can be very successfully placed in patients with either type 1 or type 2 diabetes; however, the diabetes needs to be well controlled.

Anti-coagulant therapy

Many people take anti-coagulant medications such as warfarin. These patients need careful management of their anti-coagulant therapy during the implant surgery stage. Usually we need to consult and liaise with their physicians.

Pregnancy

An elective surgical procedure is not usually recommended during pregnancy. It is best to wait until after the pregnancy to have implant surgery.

Cardiovascular disease and heart problems

Most patients with heart problems can have implant surgery, although it would be usual to liaise with the patient's cardiologist in severe cases.

Osteoporosis

There are many studies that show no difference in implant success rates between people with osteoporosis and those without. However, there are certain medications that may affect treatment – see opposite.

Bisphosphonate medication

This is a medication given to patients with osteoporosis and it is used in the treatment of some cancers that invade the bone. Bisphosphonate drugs alter bone healing. For most patients who have been taking oral bisphosphonate, and who have no complications after teeth removal, implant treatment is possible. Patients who have had intravenous bisphosphonate therapy, however, are regarded as very high risk.

Cancer treatments

Many patients are now thankfully living longer and surviving cancer thanks to an ever-growing number of new drug regimens and techniques. It is not sensible, however, to embark on any elective surgery while undergoing cancer treatment since these treatments are designed to alter the immune system. Many patients can have implant therapy after cancer treatment. The only reason you may not be able to have implants is if you have had radiotherapy to your jaws.

Factors that may rule out dental implants

There are few factors or medical conditions that make dental implant treatment inadvisable.

Some form of implant treatment is possible for most people.

As mentioned in the previous chapter, intravenous bisphosphonate therapy and radiotherapy to the jaws precludes patients from having dental implant treatment.

We also take the following into consideration:

- pregnancy or cancer therapy may mean deferring implant treatment
- age can be an issue too, although you are never too old for implant treatment – the oldest patient I have treated was 96! If you are fit enough to have minor surgery, you are fit enough for dental implant treatment
- you can, however, be too young for dental implant treatment. Dental implants can be placed only when facial growth is complete. If an implant is placed in a child, it will not move when the rest of the face develops and grows and will create cosmetic and functional issues. This means we have to wait for facial growth to be complete before implants can be used to replace missing teeth – usually around 16 to 18 years of age. Missing teeth that are planned for future replacement must be carefully managed to ensure adequate space is maintained until the patient is old enough to receive implants.

The dental implant process at Elmsleigh House

Elmsleigh House Dental Clinic is a private and referral dental clinic in Farnham, Surrey, established more than 30 years ago. Over this time, our experienced implant team has placed thousands of dental implants with natural-looking and long-lasting results. Because of our experience and outstanding results, over 500 dentists refer their patients to us for dental implants and other complex treatments. We also run regular courses to share our knowledge and expertise with other dentists.

If you are about to lose one or more teeth, or have lost teeth in the past and want a better solution than you currently have, you can discuss your concerns with the experienced implant team at Elmsleigh House.

The Advantage Implant Consult™

Whether you book-in directly to see us, or have been referred to us by your dentist for dental implants, your first appointment at Elmsleigh House is our unique Advantage Implant Consult™. During this hour-long appointment, one of our experienced implant surgeons will take the time to get to know you, listen to your concerns and discuss what you want to achieve. You will be asked questions about your overall health, and any medications that you

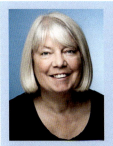

> I would like to thank Tim and the team for transforming my wife's teeth over the last 15 months or so. The improvements he made has enhanced her confidence. The quality of service was exceptional from all the staff.
>
> Tim was very friendly, sympathetic to our concerns and ensured the end quality was excellent. I often sat in the waiting room whilst my wife was being treated and was very impressed at the levels of customer service given to ALL the patients who came in.
>
> If only all businesses treated their customers like that! From this experience we can thoroughly recommend the practice to anyone looking for exceptional levels of care and high quality of treatment.
>
> Mr Williams on behalf of his wife, Gill, Surrey

have been prescribed, to ensure that everything is taken into consideration for your successful long-term implant treatment.

We will assess your whole mouth to make sure it is healthy and free from tooth decay, gum disease or other infections, and we will consider any cosmetic and functional problems. All these issues are important to the success of your dental implant treatment.

Your jaw bone and gum health will be assessed. We will look for any bone loss or gum shrinkage and whether there are any anatomical issues. In the upper jaw we are primarily concerned about the position of the maxillary sinuses (see page 16), nerves and nasal cavities. We will also pay particular attention to the position of the dental nerve that travels through your lower jaw.

X-ray pictures will be taken to assess these factors. These may be small, individual x-rays, scanning x-rays or cross-sectional ones. We use low-dose digital x-ray systems so we can assess your condition immediately and show it to you right away. We will also take digital colour photographs of your mouth and your smile to help you better understand what is happening in your mouth.

We will discuss all the treatment options, including any sedation options, that are available to you, together with the benefits, timings and fees, so you can make an informed choice about your treatment. We will answer any questions, and advise you on the solution that would best suit you, taking your health, cosmetic and financial needs into consideration.

Once agreed, your treatment solution will be written up and sent to you as your personal Dental Implant Treatment Plan. It will set out in detail:

- all stages of your treatment
- the timing of appointments
- the fees at each stage of treatment
- the Elmsleigh House guarantee and warranty review.

We guarantee these fees will not change throughout your treatment, so that you know what to expect, that you will be satisfied with your treatment and that there will be no financial surprises.

The First Stage – Initial preparatory work

It is essential that the health of your mouth, and your general health, is good before embarking on any dental implant treatment. If not, your dental implants may not osseointegrate with your jaw bone or may fail prematurely as a result of infection. Preparatory work may therefore be needed to get your mouth healthy for implant treatment.

Examples of preparatory work include:

- removal or treatment of any damaged or infected teeth
- treating gum disease, dental decay and dental infections
- having a bone or gum graft to rebuild lost tissue to enable implants to be placed
- bone grafting into your sinuses to enable implant placement in your upper jaw.

Depending on your Dental Implant Treatment Plan, which is unique to you and your dental health, implants may be placed at the same time as some preparatory work – otherwise, we may need to allow specific healing times before we can place your dental implants.

The Second Stage – Implant surgery

Dental implant surgery typically involves two minor surgical operations:

- a first operation to fit the titanium implant in your jaw bone, where it is typically buried under the gum to allow the bone to grow onto the implant over the next few months – osseointegration
- a second operation to uncover and test your implant and place a healing cap on it, which protrudes through the gum.

When people have sufficient good-quality bone and gum, it is possible to combine placing an implant and a healing cap in one operation. This speeds up treatment and helps to reduce costs, and we try to do this whenever possible. Temporary teeth are always adjusted and refitted at these operations so you have no visible gaps.

Sometimes it is also possible to place an implant and a temporary tooth or bridge in one process, which is known as 'immediate loaded teeth'. Your Dental Implant Treatment Plan will detail the timing of the stages that are specific to your bespoke treatment.

For most people, surgery is carried out under local anaesthesia (only the immediate area is made numb). For more-nervous patients we offer a range of sedation options to complement local anaesthesia, including inhalation sedation ('gas and air'), oral sedation and intravenous sedation (see page 26).

As with operations performed in hospital, all our surgical procedures are carried out under sterile operating-theatre conditions, because we believe this is vital for success.

The Third Stage – Final restorative implant work

The timing of your implant restorative work will be detailed in your treatment plan – in most cases it begins two to eight weeks after the implant osseointegration has been checked and the healing cap is placed. This allows time for the gum to heal.

An impression of the top of your implant is taken so that our dental technicians can design and construct in the laboratory your bespoke dental implant post and the cosmetic crown that will be attached to it. Depending on your individual needs, this could be a cosmetic crown, a fixed or removable bridge or an implant-stabilised removable denture.

The dental technicians will create bespoke cosmetic solutions that are custom-made using a combination of precious metals, titanium and natural-looking ceramics. With these materials, great care is taken to match the precise shape, colour and translucency of your other teeth, so that no one will know that you have replacement teeth. If you are also missing gum, it is possible to have gum-coloured porcelain or plastics added to achieve a more natural result.

If you came to us as a referred patient, your own suitably-trained dentist may be able to perform your restorative treatment.

Long-term care

To ensure your dental implants remain secure and long-lasting, you will be shown how to look after your dental implant restoration at home. You will need to visit your dentist and hygienist for regular check-ups – they will advise you on the best brushing and cleaning techniques to keep your dental implants and your mouth healthy.

Warranty review

We see all of our patients one year after treatment for a warranty review to make sure everything is healthy and functioning well with their implant.

How to contact Elmsleigh House

To book your Advantage Implant Consult™ appointment at Elmsleigh House Dental Clinic or to find out more information:

Telephone the Welcome Team on 01252 713797

Email us at info@elmsleighhouse.co.uk

Visit our website at **www.elmsleighhouse.co.uk**

Elmsleigh House Dental Clinic,
6 Station Hill, Farnham, Surrey GU9 8AA

Questions for your implant consultation